OTHER WORKS BY GRAND MASTER NAN LU

*Digesting the Universe: A Revolutionary Framework
for Healthy Metabolism Function*

*A Revolutionary Framework for Using Modern Science
and Ancient Wisdom for Breast Cancer Prevention*

Ask Dr. Lu

*Traditional Chinese Medicine: A Natural Guide
to Weight Loss That Lasts*

*Traditional Chinese Medicine: A Woman's Guide
to a Trouble-Free Menopause*

*Traditional Chinese Medicine: A Woman's Guide
to Healing from Breast Cancer*

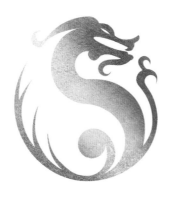

DRAGON'S
WAY
QIGONG®

BY GRAND MASTER NAN LU

WEEKLY GUIDE

Dragon's Way Qigong® Weekly Guide

First paperback edition published in 2020 by Tao of Healing Publishing.

For information, contact Tao of Healing Publishing:
Tao of Healing
34 West 27th Street, Suite 1212
New York, NY 10001
www.taoofhealing.com

Library of Congress Catalog-in-Publication Data has been applied for:
ISBN: 978-0-9845508-1-4

The material in this book is for educational purposes only. Since each person's circumstance is unique, we recommend consulting your healthcare practitioner with respect to your particular medical condition. The use of this material is the sole responsibility of the user and at his or her discretion. The authors and publisher disclaim any responsibility for the liability, loss or risk, personal or otherwise, which is incurred as a consequence, directly or indirectly, of the use and/or application of any of the contents of this work.

CONTENTS

A MESSAGE FROM GRAND MASTER NAN LU 6

INTRODUCTION. 8

WEEK 1: EVERYTHING IS ENERGY. 20

WEEK 2: LIVER/GALLBLADDER. 32

WEEK 3: KIDNEY/BLADDER. 48

WEEK 4: SPLEEN/STOMACH 64

WEEK 5: LUNG/LARGE INTESTINE 80

WEEK 6: HEART/SMALL INTESTINE 96

WHAT IS QIGONG?. 112

QIGONG MOVEMENTS. 116

EATING-FOR-HEALING 126

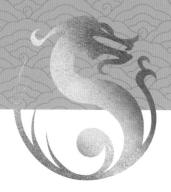

WELCOME TO DRAGON'S WAY QIGONG®. This journey will change your life and the relationship you have with your body forever. My approach is based on a system that understands the body's ability to heal itself. I will teach you how to apply that innate healing gift to all areas of your life.

True change is possible if you understand that everything is energy and everything is connected. Energy is the body's life force. The body constantly uses all of its resources to maintain balance. When you are off-balance, you may begin to notice physical symptoms, weight fluctuations or emotional highs and lows. During your Dragon's Way Qigong experience, I will help you learn how to increase your energy and use it to create better health.

For thousands of years, the Chinese culture has known how to access the wisdom of Universal energy by following Natural Law. This law is not a theory. It was not developed by the human mind. It is something much larger than you or me. Natural Law offers us a framework to understand the cooperative relationships inherent in all living things.

GRAND MASTER NAN LU

Billions of people in the Chinese culture have used traditional Chinese medicine (TCM) to thrive. TCM has sustained an entire civilization over millennia because it honors the body's innate ability to heal by providing a road map for living in harmony with Nature. Ancient healers understood prevention as a fundamental requirement for good health. Their job was to discover the root cause of illness to bring the body back to balance. Now, more than ever, we need this system to support our increasingly stressful lifestyles.

Dragon's Way Qigong comes without side-effects—only results that allow you to experience life with a newfound sense of freedom. You will be able to handle stress differently. Your ability to regain physical, mental and emotional balance will be greatly enhanced. Your emotions and relationship with your body will change. Your cravings for certain foods will change. Your sleep patterns and level of peacefulness will change.

I will help you go beyond your current imbalances and teach you how to use your untapped energy to rediscover good health.

You have just taken the first steps toward a life-long journey of health, healing and happiness—congratulations!

Dragon's Way Qigong is built upon the profound understanding of the body's relationship to Qi, or energy. Over the course of this program, you will learn how to build your Qi and understand how to use it wisely.

This guidebook is intended to be used in conjunction with the Dragon's Way Qigong video. The video includes a teaching module and a practice module. This guide will support you through the program.

In addition to the Qigong movements, this guide invites you to make gradual changes each week to your diet and in the way you manage your energy and stress. Weekly lessons will help you tune in to the signs and signals your body is sending. At the end of 6 weeks, like thousands of other Dragon's Way Qigong participants, you will have developed a new level of personal freedom.

INTRODUCTION

If you are participating in a Dragon's Way Qigong class with a certified instructor, use this guide to record your notes and any changes that you experience. If you are interested in delving deeper into traditional Chinese medicine theories, refer to *TCM: A Natural Guide to Weight Loss That Lasts.*

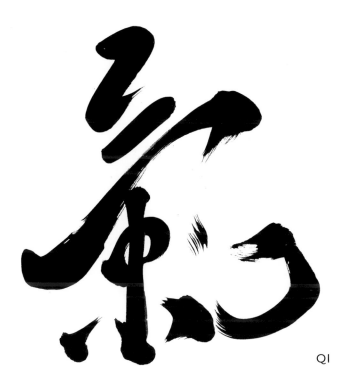

QI

WU MING QIGONG PRACTICE

In Dragon's Way Qigong, you will learn 10 *Wu Ming* Qigong movements, which are illustrated and explained in detail on page 116.

Qigong is an ancient energy practice that reawakens your natural healing ability and allows you to tap into the infinite wisdom of the Universe. It is one of the best ways to increase your Qi, or energy, in a gentle yet profound manner.

EATING-FOR-HEALING PLAN

Dragon's Way Qigong offers an approach to eating that goes beyond the physical properties of vitamins and nutrients to the level of essence. A food's essence is an expression of its relationship with Nature. This relation-ship contains a message that resonates deep within the body to promote a healthy balance of energy flow. On page 130, you will find a suggested eating plan and a recommended list of foods.

PROGRAM

LIFESTYLE

Everything in life—work, eating habits, activity level, emotions and your overall environment—impacts your Qi. Each week, you will learn how to understand the effects of your daily lifestyle from an energetic perspective.

We all want freedom—from health issues, from fear, from worry—but most importantly, the freedom to live a healthy, happy life. Create the life you want. Use your energy in a positive way to make your life more beautiful.

HERBAL SUPPLEMENTS

Herbs are food. They carry messages of Universal wisdom that energetically support you. TCM has been incorporating herbs into its healing plans for thousands of years. Much like the foods chosen for this program, the herbal formulas selected will help build your energy foundation and allow your Qi to move more freely. This is an optional but highly recommended component.

EVERYTHING IS ENERGY

As in many other ancient traditions, Chinese masters studied the link between man and Nature. These practitioners sat in silent meditation and observed the connections apparent in the world around them. What they discovered formed the basis of TCM and now Dragon's Way Qigong—everything is energy and all energy is consciousness.

You are an energy being. Your body is a reflection of your life. It will always show what's happening deep within on an energetic level. All life imbalances will affect the smooth flow of energy.

TCM views the body as being in a state of balance versus imbalance. Any imbalances that occur happen first on the energetic level. If not addressed, these imbalances will progress to a physical sign or symptom, such as excess weight or emotions, bloating and aches and pains, all the way to diabetes and cancers.

Symptoms are the body's way of asking for support. Maintaining the free flow of energy is the key to good health.

ABOUT QI

YOU ARE AN ENERGY BEING

All of life contains Qi. Qi is the animating force that guides you through life and determines your health and well-being.

We come into this world with a finite amount of energy that we inherit from our parents. The quality of this inherited Qi cannot be enhanced or improved. It is pre-determined by the health of our parents.

Your everyday activities, no matter how mundane, draw upon this energy source. In order to maintain health and balance, we need to continually acquire more Qi from external sources.

Learning to save your energy—and acquire more—is the key to your success with Dragon's Way Qigong. Acquiring Qi is the gift that ancient Chinese masters discovered. It's the secret to health, longevity and living life with complete freedom!

To understand energy and its relationship to your body, we turn to the Five Element Consciousness Framework.

FIVE ELEMENT CONSCIOUSNESS FRAMEWORK

Ancient masters recognized that all life—whether human, plant, animal, microbe or cosmic—is connected. This knowing led them to generate a blueprint to "see" the energetic connections in all things. They applied this deep knowing to the workings of the human body.

In this framework, each of Nature's five elements—Wood, Fire, Earth, Metal and Water—is linked to an organ system, an emotion, a color, a taste, as well as other characteristics. If one organ does not function optimally, the others compensate in an effort to restore balance.

DECODING THE BODY'S SYMPTOMS

Have you ever found yourself with an intense craving for something sour? There are no accidents!

In the Five Element Consciousness Framework, there are 5 circles with 2 partner organs listed in each. Each pair has its own responsibility to support the overall health of the body. Each also has its own way of communicating when it needs support. For example, your craving for sour foods is a signal from your Liver.

A feeling of intense worry may indicate an imbalance in your Stomach function. These messages don't necessarily indicate a problem with the physical organ; they signal an energetic imbalance. Our bodies' symptoms are calls for support; the Five Element Consciousness Framework gives us a roadmap for decoding them.

Take time to study the Five Element Consciousness Framework. Refer to it as often as possible. As you learn more about yourself in the next 6 weeks, you'll discover infinite possibilities and connections within the framework. Is there a season in which you always seem to get sick? Does a certain emotion particularly affect you? Which organ is it connected to?

Although each of the five elements has its own individual components, they are all connected into one harmonious whole. These connections are indicated by the solid and dashed lines linking each of the circles and therefore each of the organs.

The body is a microcosm of Nature.

—Grand Master Nan Lu

FIVE ELEMENT CONSO

1
2 GA
3
4 Eye
5 Tend
6 Ang

1 **KIDNEY**
2 **URINARY BLADDER**
3 **WATER**

4 Ear   7 Winter
5 Bone   8 Black
6 Fear   9 Salty

1 **LUNG**
2 **LARGE INTESTINE**
3 **METAL**

4 Nose   7 Autumn
5 Skin &   8 White
  Hair   9 Spicy
6 Grief

→ Nurturing
   Relationship

⤏ Cooperative
   Relationship

USNESS FRAMEWORK

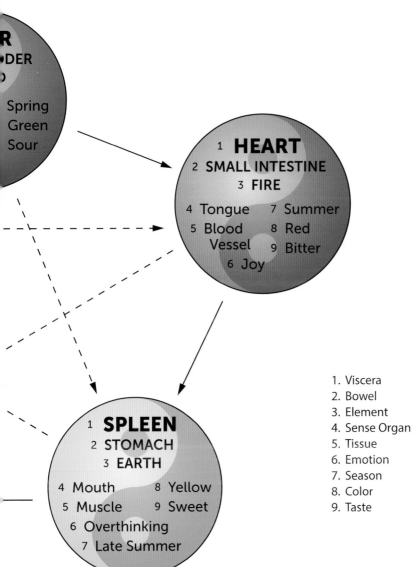

R
·DER

Spring
Green
Sour

1 **HEART**
2 **SMALL INTESTINE**
3 **FIRE**

4 Tongue   7 Summer
5 Blood   8 Red
   Vessel   9 Bitter
6 Joy

1 **SPLEEN**
2 **STOMACH**
3 **EARTH**

4 Mouth   8 Yellow
5 Muscle   9 Sweet
6 Overthinking
7 Late Summer

1. Viscera
2. Bowel
3. Element
4. Sense Organ
5. Tissue
6. Emotion
7. Season
8. Color
9. Taste

THE WEEKS AHEAD

In the 6 weeks ahead, you will begin to develop a different relationship with your body. Weekly, we will journey through the Five Element Consciousness Framework to understand the significance of each organ system and how it communicates through physical and emotional signs. You will begin to acquire Qi by practicing Qigong and following the eating-for-healing plan.

> Week 1: Preparation Week: Everything is Energy
>
> Week 2: Liver/Gallbladder
>
> Week 3: Kidney/Bladder
>
> Week 4: Spleen/Stomach
>
> Week 5: Lung/Large Intestine
>
> Week 6: Heart/Small Intestine

PROGRAM GOAL

My goal is to help you rebuild a relationship with your body through the most powerful channel—your life force. Over the next 6 weeks, you will be guided to learn how to rediscover the gifts you were born with and to feel healthy, vibrant and more balanced. Once you learn this system, it is yours to continue using for a lifetime. It will give you freedom to explore life with a newfound lightness! Let's get started.

–Grand Master Nan Lu

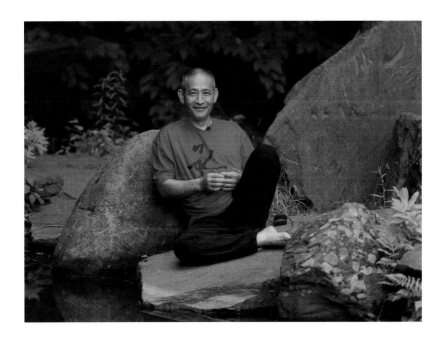

WEEK ONE AT A GLANCE

I LIKE TO REFER TO WEEK 1 AS YOUR PREPARATION WEEK. DURING THIS WEEK, I'LL GUIDE YOU TO DO THE FOLLOWING:

- Learn 4 Qigong movements to practice daily.

- Gradually eliminate bread, meat and dairy from your diet.

- Begin to analyze some of your lifestyle choices and your current state of health through the provided self-assessments.

- Slowly incorporate suggested lifestyle changes.

WEEK 1

EVERYETHING
IS ENERGY

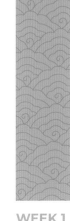

"YOUR LIFE BELONGS TO THE
UNIVERSE; YOUR HEALTH
BELONGS TO YOU."

- Nei Jing, ancient Chinese medical text

WHAT BALANCED QI LOOKS LIKE:

- BALANCED
  EMOTIONS

- BALANCED WEIGHT

- HEALTHY DIGESTION

- PEACEFUL SLEEP

- SENSE OF CALM

- CREATIVE

- ENERGIZED

PREPARING TO BUILD QI
QI IS ALL AROUND US

Everything is energy, and all energy has purpose. Once you accumulate energy, your body has the wisdom to use it wisely for self-healing. But where do you get it from? You can't buy it. Energy—Qi—is priceless! Luckily it's all around us and available 24 hours a day.

So if Qi is all around us, how do we access it? The good news is, there are many ways! You can aquire Qi through consistent Dragon's Way Qigong practice, following the eating-for-healing plan, taking the herbal supplements and spending time in Nature, to name a few. This week bring your awareness within. How do you use your Qi? How do you spend it? Jot some notes below.

OBSERVE YOUR LIFESTYLE

No matter what activity you engage in, you use energy. Read the list below and check yes or no to answer each statement.

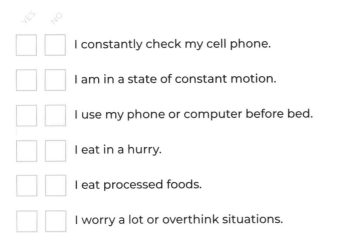

YES NO

☐ ☐ I constantly check my cell phone.

☐ ☐ I am in a state of constant motion.

☐ ☐ I use my phone or computer before bed.

☐ ☐ I eat in a hurry.

☐ ☐ I eat processed foods.

☐ ☐ I worry a lot or overthink situations.

How many times did you answer yes? Stop wasting your energy! Here are my suggestions for creating new patterns:

Turn off your cell phone after 8 p.m.

Take 5-minute WiFi breaks once an hour.

Go for a walk, sit quietly or listen to music.

Eat in a quiet, peaceful environment.

When a worrisome thought comes to mind, change your thinking to see that everything happens for good.

ENERGY INVENTORY

NOTICE HOW YOU FEEL

Pay attention to your body's messages. Take some time to notice how you feel. Check off anything that applies to you now. Return to this page after 6 weeks to track your progress.

BEFORE AFTER

BEFORE AFTER

☐ ☐ Angry moods

☐ ☐ Fatigue

☐ ☐ Anxiety

☐ ☐ Food allergies

☐ ☐ Arthritic conditions

☐ ☐ Forgetfulness

☐ ☐ Bloating

☐ ☐ Frequent urination

☐ ☐ Bone loss

☐ ☐ Headaches

☐ ☐ Cold hands and feet

☐ ☐ High blood pressure

☐ ☐ Constipation

☐ ☐ High cholesterol

☐ ☐ Diarrhea

☐ ☐ Hot flashes

☐ ☐ Dizziness

☐ ☐ Insomnia

	BEFORE	AFTER			BEFORE	AFTER	
	☐	☐	Joint pain		☐	☐	Prostate issues
	☐	☐	Knee and heel pain		☐	☐	Ringing in the ears
	☐	☐	Lack of sexual desire		☐	☐	Skin rashes
	☐	☐	Lower back pain		☐	☐	Stomachaches
	☐	☐	Menstrual difficulties		☐	☐	Stress
	☐	☐	Mood swings		☐	☐	Thyroid issues
	☐	☐	Muscle tension		☐	☐	_____
	☐	☐	Palpitations		☐	☐	_____

$E= MC^2$

Energy is meant to flow smoothly. When energy flows, the body is balanced and healthy. When energy gets stuck, the body expresses physical and emotional symptoms. Energy and mass are interchangeable.

ACTION PLAN

1. QIGONG PRACTICE: CREATING FLOW

Just as you take a shower to clean the outside of your body, we'll use Qigong to clean the inside. Start slowly by learning 4 movements this week. Turn to the Qigong section and practice movements 1–3 and number 10:

1. The Dragon's Toe Dance

2. The Dragon Kicks Forward

3. The Dragon's Twist

10. The Dragon Stands Between Heaven and Earth

2. EATING-FOR-HEALING PLAN

When you eat, the body uses Qi to digest and process food. This week, reduce foods that require large amounts of Qi to digest. What you save will be used by the body for self-healing.

Begin the week by reducing and ultimately eliminating the following heavy foods: bread, meat and dairy. Coffee and tea are fine, as is an occasional glass of wine.

Spend some extra time in the produce aisle this week. What foods are you drawn to? The tastes you crave will give you insight into what your body really needs. If you're craving something that's not on the suggested list, go for it. But enjoy every bite. This is not a diet of restriction but rather an eating plan that embraces fresh, light foods.

GUIDELINES:

- Eat until you are 70-80% full.
- Eat your heaviest meals early in the day.
- Eliminate raw vegetables and iced drinks.

Turn to the eating-for-healing section on page 126 and review the suggested foods and sample menus.

3. LIFESTYLE TIPS

How are you using your Qi? Become aware of your daily habits, such as: how long you spend on your cell phone or computer, what time you head to bed and how you react to stressful situations.

4. HERBAL SUPPLEMENTS

If you've decided to include herbal supplements, begin taking 3 tablets of Imperial Qi and 3 tablets of Green Dragon each morning and each evening with warm water.

Other supplements or medications should be taken 30 minutes before or after your herbs. If you forget to take your herbs in the morning, simply leave 6 hours between the morning and evening doses.

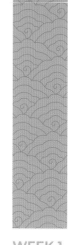

CLOSING WORDS FOR WEEK 1

Before you begin Week 2, make some observations about your first week. As your body begins to shift, become more aware of the changes taking place. Your body is your loyal friend. It will always do its best to support you. When it needs energetic help, it will send you messages through signs and symptoms. What are you noticing?

DID YOU KNOW?

Picture the body as an organic whole with many moving parts. All parts of the body—muscle, organ, blood and energetic frequencies—continually work together to allow it to function at the highest level possible.

WEEK 1
JOURNAL

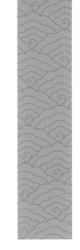

WEEK 1
JOURNAL

WEEK 1
JOURNAL

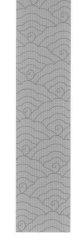

WEEK TWO AT A GLANCE

DURING WEEK 2, I'LL INTRODUCE YOU TO A NEW WAY OF UNDERSTANDING YOUR BODY USING THE FIVE ELEMENT CONSCIOUSNESS FRAMEWORK. WE WILL BEGIN WITH THE LIVER AND GALLBLADDER PARTNERSHIP. IN ADDITION, I'LL GUIDE YOU TO DO THE FOLLOWING:

· Learn 2 additional Qigong movements, for a total of 6 to practice daily.

· Prepare suggested foods that support the Liver and Gallbladder.

· Assess your level of stress and apply the provided tips.

IT'S ALL
ABOUT THE LIVER

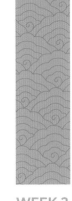

DO YOU WANT TO BE LIKE THE
CAT THAT IS STRONG, AGILE AND
FLEXIBLE, OR LIKE THE COW
WHICH HAS HUGE MUSCLES BUT
LITTLE STRENGTH?

–Grand Master Nan Lu

LIVER HIGHLIGHTS

PARTNER ORGAN:
Gallbladder

EMOTION:
Anger

ELEMENT:
Wood

SEASON:
Spring

SENSE ORGAN:
Eye

COLOR:
Green

TISSUE ORGAN:
Tendon

TASTE:
Sour

STARTING THE WEEK

You're about to begin Week 2. How are you feeling? Remember, symptoms are the body's way of talking to you. If you are following the program consistently, you're beginning to break down internal "garbage." Circle any changes that you have noticed since you started the program.

More energized . . . . Less energized

Bigger appetite . . . . Smaller appetite

Emotional balance . . . . Mood swings

More peaceful . . . . About the same

Fewer body aches . . . . . . About the same

Other _____

THE IMPORTANCE OF THE LIVER

We live in fast-paced times. Many of us are constantly in motion. For the body to keep up with this pace, Liver energy must be strong and flow freely. The Liver plays a key role in helping the body manage stress on a daily basis. Healthy Liver function is so important that it is the focal point of the whole Dragon's Way Qigong program.

A hectic lifestyle, along with mental and physical stress, causes different degrees of Liver function disorder. When your body is calm, its inner vibration has an even tone. But stress and anger create imbalances in the body. Emotions upset the smooth flow of Liver Qi. This, in turn, prevents the Liver from functioning optimally.

WHAT THE LIVER CAN DO

The Liver is known as the "go with the flow" organ. The Liver and its partner organ, the Gallbladder, are responsible for the smooth flow of blood, Qi and emotions in the body. Their cooperative relationship with the Spleen and the Stomach results in a healthy digestive system. Healthy Liver function is also evident in physical and emotional flexibility and healthy eyes, hair and nails.

The Liver is the main organ responsible for women's health. Keeping Liver Qi flowing smoothly is the key to normal menstrual cycles, reproductive health and breast health.

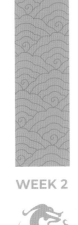

WEEKLY GOAL

Stress puts an added strain on your Liver. My goal this week is to help you become aware of these energy drains. How can you slow down? Where can you cut back on your stress?

—Grand Master Nan Lu

WHAT DOES IT LOOK LIKE WHEN THE LIVER/GALLBLADDER DOES NOT FLOW SMOOTHLY?

- Stress
- Angry moods
- PMS, menopause
- Infertility
- Dry and brittle nails
- Cold hands and feet
- Burning or irritation of the eyes
- Migraine headaches
- Arthritic conditions
- Tendon issues
- Indigestion and bloating
- High cholesterol

TUNE INWARD

What foods are you craving? Write them here. Throughout this week, become aware of the foods and tastes your body asks for.

_____   _____

_____   _____

_____   _____

_____   _____

FIVE ELEMENT CONSCIOUSNESS FRAMEWORK

1. Viscera
2. Bowel
3. Element
4. Sense Organ
5. Tissue
6. Emotion
7. Season
8. Color
9. Taste

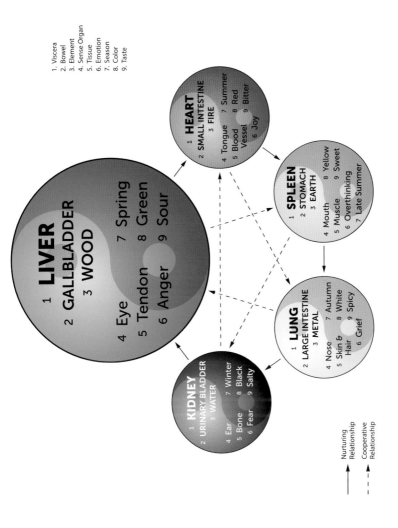

LIVER
1 LIVER
2 GALLBLADDER
3 WOOD
4 Eye
5 Tendon
6 Anger
7 Spring
8 Green
9 Sour

HEART
1 HEART
2 SMALL INTESTINE
3 FIRE
4 Tongue
5 Blood Vessel
6 Joy
7 Summer
8 Red
9 Bitter

SPLEEN
1 SPLEEN
2 STOMACH
3 EARTH
4 Mouth
5 Muscle
6 Overthinking
7 Late Summer
8 Yellow
9 Sweet

LUNG
1 LUNG
2 LARGE INTESTINE
3 METAL
4 Nose
5 Skin & Hair
6 Grief
7 Autumn
8 White
9 Spicy

KIDNEY
1 KIDNEY
2 URINARY BLADDER
3 WATER
4 Ear
5 Bone
6 Fear
7 Winter
8 Black
9 Salty

Nurturing Relationship

Cooperative Relationship

RELATIONSHIPS

The Liver and Gallbladder help to move Qi, blood, bile and fat through the body. The Gallbladder is also your master decision maker. This duo supports your emotional and physical flexibility.

ELEMENT: WOOD

The Wood element is related to the Liver. Its nature is to move freely, like the branches of a tree. Just as trees gracefully dance in the wind, allow your body to follow Nature's energy flow. Don't just sit there—get up and move. Dance!

SENSE ORGAN: EYES

The eyes are the sense organs related to the Liver. Cues that your Liver Qi is imbalanced include watery, itchy eyes (especially during Spring), blurry vision, floaters, a change in vision and red, dry or itchy eyes.

TISSUE ORGAN: TENDON

TCM believes that strength comes from the tendons, not the muscles. Ultimate flexibility—in emotions and in the physical body—is a sign of balanced Liver Qi.

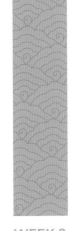

EMOTION: ANGER

Liver energy loves to go with the flow. If Liver Qi is not flowing, it will communicate with you through excess anger and frustration.

SEASON: SPRING

The Spring season is the symbol of activity and rebirth. During this time of year, Nature begins to reemerge. This energy is vibrant and active, and must be free-flowing. If your body cannot match the season's energy, you may experience seasonal allergies.

COLOR: GREEN

Are you drawn to one color over another? It's no surprise that the color green resonates with the Liver. After all, all of Nature turns green in Spring! Give your Liver a boost by wearing green. Take a walk in Nature and become more aware of your surroundings.

TASTE: SOUR

Pucker up! Sour foods energetically support Liver function. To give this organ system a boost, squeeze a lemon over your cooked vegetables or try some pickled foods.

THE BODY NEVER LIES

MESSAGES FROM YOUR LIVER

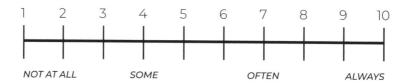

NOT AT ALL   SOME   OFTEN   ALWAYS

Begin to see yourself. On a scale from 1–10, how would you rate your:

- Stress levels
- Tendency to become easily angered
- Physical flexibility
- Emotional flexibility
- Ability to let go of things or feelings that no longer serve you

DID YOU KNOW?

Emotions are the root cause of 99% of all health issues. In a constant state of push and pull, emotions can challenge the body's well-being.

YOUR WEEKLY
ACTION PLAN

1. QIGONG PRACTICE: CREATING FLOW

Turn to the Qigong section. During this week, you'll be learning 2 additional movements. Practice the entire set at least once per day.

1. The Dragon's Toe Dance

2. The Dragon Kicks Forward

3. The Dragon's Twist

4. The Dragon's Punch

5. The Dragon Looks at Its Tail

10. The Dragon Stands Between Heaven and Earth

WEEKLY CHALLENGE

Increase your Q! Hold Number 10 for 8 minutes or longer.

–Grand Master Nan Lu

2. EATING-FOR-HEALING PLAN

By now you've reduced or eliminated bread, meat and dairy in your diet. Continue to become familiar with the eating plan. Experiment with new recipes on our website: tcmworld.org/health/recipes. Eat seasonal foods that are organic or locally grown and remember to cook vegetables; warm foods will aid your body in the digestive process.

When following the eating-for-healing plan, include some of these foods to further support your Liver function:

Bamboo shoots	Lemon
Bee pollen	Pickled ginger
Broccoli rabe	Plums
Dandelion greens	Scallions
Eggplant	Sour pickles
Fennel	Vinegar
Green apples	Mung beans

DID YOU KNOW?

The Dragon's Toe Dance helps to stimulate Liver energy. It's also an easy movement to practice while waiting for the bus or standing in line at the market. If your body is sending messages of Liver imbalance, add an extra practice daily.

3. LIFESTYLE TIPS

1. Think of the many ways you rely on your eyes throughout the day. Give your Liver some added support—turn off your computer and cell phone each evening. This will also help to reduce the electromagnetic fields (EMFs) that your Liver works so hard to process.

2. Recognize yourself as an energetic being. Your feelings are energy, your emotions are energy—everything is energy. Begin to see and understand that this energy is all around you.

3. Relax and release your stress. When you feel stressed, you often grind your teeth and clench your fists. The body tightens and everything becomes rigid. When you finally release stress through crying or screaming, the body begins to loosen. This relaxed feeling is Liver Qi in motion!

TRY THIS EXERCISE:
BREAK EGGS!

Breaking eggs is a great way to release your pent-up stress and frustration. Exercise your emotional flexibility by throwing eggs in the woods.

CLOSING WORDS FOR WEEK 2

Throughout this week, keep a log of your Qigong practice. Make quality practice your priority. The more you practice, the better your results will be.

Evaluate your level of stress and take a step toward relieving a stressful situation. Revisit page 43 for some suggestions.

And finally, be good to yourself. Find whatever time you can to relax, unwind and reconnect with Nature. Begin to reawaken the understanding that your body has the powerful ability to reach a higher level of health.

_____

_____

_____

MAKE THIS YOUR MANTRA:

There are no accidents.

Everything is happening for a reason.

Everything is happening for good.

How can I see the good?

—Grand Master Nan Lu

WEEK 2
JOURNAL

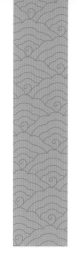

WEEK 2
JOURNAL

WEEK 2
JOURNAL

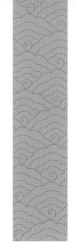

WEEK THREE AT A GLANCE

DURING WEEK 3, YOU'LL LEARN HOW TO
RELATE TO THE KIDNEY AND BLADDER
FROM A FIVE ELEMENT CONSCIOUSNESS
FRAMEWORK. IN ADDITION, I'LL GUIDE YOU
TO DO THE FOLLOWING:

WEEK 3

- Learn 2 additional Qigong movements, for a total of 8 to practice daily.

- Prepare suggested foods that support
  the Kidney and Bladder.

- Understand how and why saving Qi
  can lead to a balanced lifestyle.

THE KIDNEY
YOUR ENERGY TANK

THINK OF YOUR LIFE AS A CANDLE.
SOME CANDLES ARE SMALL,
SOME ARE LARGE. HOW WISELY
YOU BURN YOUR FLAME WILL
DETERMINE HOW WELL YOU LIVE
YOUR LIFE.

–Grand Master Nan Lu

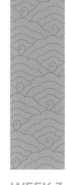

WEEK 3

KIDNEY HIGHLIGHTS

PARTNER ORGAN:
Urinary Bladder

EMOTION:
Fear

ELEMENT:
Water

SEASON:
Winter

SENSE ORGAN:
Ear

COLOR:
Black or
Dark Blue

TISSUE ORGAN:
Bone

TASTE:
Salty

STARTING THE WEEK

You're about to begin Week 3. Have you noticed any physical or emotional changes thus far? Is your Qigong practice becoming a daily habit? Use this chart to track your practice and note how you feel afterward.

	MORNING	EVENING	EXTRA	NOTES
Sunday	☐	☐	☐	_____
Monday	☐	☐	☐	_____
Tuesday	☐	☐	☐	_____
Wednesday	☐	☐	☐	_____
Thursday	☐	☐	☐	_____
Friday	☐	☐	☐	_____
Saturday	☐	☐	☐	_____

THE IMPORTANCE OF THE KIDNEY

The second organ of importance during the Dragon's Way Qigong program is the Kidney. The Kidney is associated with all of your body's Qi and genetic wisdom.

The role of the Kidney is vital; it holds the key to longevity and intelligence, and stores all of the Qi you inherit at birth.

After you're born, your body uses your inherited Qi for growth. All growth, including teeth, bones, sexual development, hormones and the ability to reproduce are related to the quality and quantity of Kidney Qi. Learning how to use this Qi wisely will help you stay strong and powerful throughout your entire life.

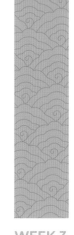

WHAT THE KIDNEY CAN DO

The Kidney and Bladder are considered partners. Together these organs manage the power to access the best of your genetic code and provide support to the Heart. Strong Qi is your secret to anti-aging and combating issues like fatigue, memory loss, bone loss and anxiety.

WEEKLY GOAL

Imagine that the Qi you've inherited is inside a deep well. You draw from it wisely, taking Qi only when needed. Because you didn't waste your Qi, you have a good amount remaining by the time you reach your 50s. You will continue to enjoy a long, healthy life. My goal this week is to help you see your Qi inheritance in this manner. How can you conserve what you've been given?

–Grand Master Nan Lu

WHAT DOES IT LOOK LIKE WHEN THE KIDNEY/BLADDER DOES NOT FLOW SMOOTHLY?

- Hair loss

- Bone pain, low bone density, broken bones

- Forgetfulness, memory loss

- Knee and heel pain

- Chronic lower back pain

- Ringing in the ears

- Fear, anxiety, panic attacks

- Dental problems

- Pain in the bottom of the feet

- Thyroid problems

- Frequent urination, waking to urinate

- Prostate and sexual function problems

- Insomnia

- Hot flashes

- High blood pressure

TUNE INWARD

Which of your daily activities zap your energy? Write them here. Throughout this week, become aware of your energy leaks.

_____ _____

_____ _____

FIVE ELEMENT CONSCIOUSNESS FRAMEWORK

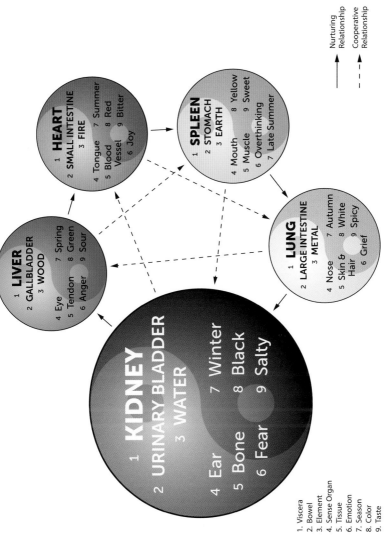

HEART
2 SMALL INTESTINE
3 FIRE
4 Tongue   7 Summer
5 Blood   8 Red
   Vessel   9 Bitter
6 Joy

SPLEEN
2 STOMACH
3 EARTH
4 Mouth   8 Yellow
5 Muscle   9 Sweet
6 Overthinking
7 Late Summer

LIVER
2 GALLBLADDER
3 WOOD
   7 Spring
4 Eye   8 Green
5 Tendon 9 Sour
6 Anger

LUNG
2 LARGE INTESTINE
3 METAL
4 Nose   7 Autumn
5 Skin & 8 White
   Hair   9 Spicy
6 Grief

KIDNEY
2 URINARY BLADDER
3 WATER
4 Ear   7 Winter
5 Bone   8 Black
6 Fear   9 Salty

1. Viscera
2. Bowel
3. Element
4. Sense Organ
5. Tissue
6. Emotion
7. Season
8. Color
9. Taste

⟶ Nurturing Relationship

- - ⟶ Cooperative Relationship

WEEK 3

RELATIONSHIPS

The Kidney and Bladder are partner organs. They work in harmony to support the body. This is especially true for men's health. Together, they play a major role in maintaining a sharp mind and good memory.

ELEMENT: WATER

The Water element is related to the Kidney. Water is powerful and unstoppable.

SENSE ORGAN: EAR

The ears are the outer organ that connect to the Kidney. Protect the ears from cold winter winds with a hat or earmuffs.

TISSUE ORGAN: BONE

Your Kidney Qi is associated with your bones and teeth. Kidney Qi naturally declines as you age. Many elderly people have brittle bones that break easily. Many also have tooth decay or loss. Can you see the connection?

EMOTION: FEAR

Emotions are the body's way of communicating. Approaching emotions as signs allows you to understand your body from an energetic perspective. For people who experience fear on a regular basis, the body is simply saying that the Kidney needs energetic support.

SEASON: WINTER

The Winter season is associated with the Kidney. Think about what happens in Nature during Winter—birds fly south, animals hibernate and plants go dormant. This deep restorative period allows for rebirth in Spring. As human beings, we too need time to pull back and recharge. The quality of your energy during Winter will determine how smoothly you transition into Spring.

COLOR: BLACK OR DARK BLUE

The colors black and dark blue resonate with the Kidney. If you find yourself wearing these colors often, congratulate yourself! You are beginning to listen to your body.

TASTE: SALTY

The taste that directly impacts the Kidney is salt. Shellfish that live in salty ocean waters are beneficial to the Kidney, as are bone soups.

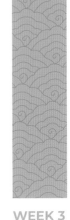

THE BODY NEVER LIES

MESSAGES FROM YOUR KIDNEY

Are you now more aware of how energy leaks affect your body? Reflect on the ways in which you waste Qi. Write them in the box below. What are you doing to acquire Qi?

Waste Qi	Acquire Qi

DID YOU KNOW?

Fear is based on the past. Somewhere in your consciousness, you're holding on to the memory of something that frightened you. This event may have directly impacted you or may have been something that you experienced indirectly. Why live in the past? What might happen if you release that fear? Trust that life is unfolding exactly as intended. There are no accidents.

YOUR WEEKLY

ACTION PLAN

1. QIGONG PRACTICE: CREATING FLOW

Turn to the Qigong section. Practice movements 1–7 and 10 at least once per day, holding number 10 for 8 minutes or longer.

1. The Dragon's Toe Dance

2. The Dragon Kicks Forward

3. The Dragon's Twist

4. The Dragon's Punch

5. The Dragon Looks at Its Tail

6. The Dragon Taps Its Foot

7. Rocking the Baby Dragon

10. The Dragon Stands Between Heaven and Earth

WEEKLY CHALLENGE

Add an additional practice of number 10 every day this week.

–Grand Master Nan Lu

2. EATING-FOR-HEALING PLAN

When following the eating-for-healing plan, include some of these foods to further support your Kidney function:

Shellfish (shrimp, squid, lobster, clams)

Bone soup

Walnuts

Pine nuts

Cauliflower

Seaweed

Black sesame seeds (black tahini)

Sunflower seeds

Black beans

Bean curd

Walnut oil

Sesame oil

Cinnamon

Cloves

DID YOU KNOW?

You can impact your Kidney meridian through a point at the bottom of your foot. So, what's the best way to stimulate this meridian? Roll a tennis ball under each foot for 5 minutes at a time.

3. LIFESTYLE TIPS

1. Winter is a time of deep rest. Nurture yourself! Support your Kidney energy by taking frequent breaks throughout the day and heading to bed before midnight.

2. Have you noticed that walnuts look like little brains? Walnuts are a warming food that support Kidney Qi. The Kidney supports the brain and the bones, and provides energetic support to the entire body. Try this recipe:

Walnut and Black Sesame Seed Snacks

1/4 lb walnuts
1/4 lb black sesame seeds
2 oz honey

Grind the walnuts and sesame seeds in a food processor. Steam in a double boiler for 1 hour.

Remove from the heat and mix in the honey. When cool, shape the mixture into balls. Place on waxed paper and refrigerate until firm.

4. HERBAL SUPPLEMENTS

Continue taking Green Dragon and Imperial Qi twice daily. For additional support, add Swimming Dragon to your routine. Take 2 tablets each morning and each evening with warm water.

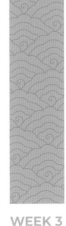

CLOSING WORDS FOR WEEK 3

During this week, you may find your energy shifting. Things that once bothered you may not be as important to you now. You may be losing weight and experiencing a burst of energy. The opposite may also be true. As you acquire more Qi, the body's wisdom begins to wake up. Continue and remember—the more you practice, the better your results will be.

Before you begin Week 4, make some observations about your third week. What have you noticed?

_____

_____

_____

Qigong is the ultimate healing journey. The answer lies within.

–Grand Master Nan Lu

WEEK 3
JOURNAL

_____

_____

_____

_____

_____

_____

_____

_____

_____

_____

_____

_____

_____

_____

_____

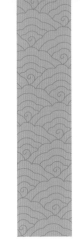

JOURNAL

WEEK 3
JOURNAL

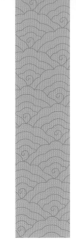

WEEK FOUR AT A GLANCE

DURING WEEK 4, YOU'LL LEARN HOW TRADITIONAL CHINESE MEDICINE VIEWS CERTAIN ASPECTS OF THE SPLEEN AND STOMACH RELATIONSHIP, ACCORDING TO THE FIVE ELEMENT CONSCIOUSNESS FRAMEWORK. IN ADDITION, I'LL GUIDE YOU TO DO THE FOLLOWING:

- Learn 2 additional Qigong movements, for a total of 10 to practice daily.

- Prepare suggested foods that support the Spleen and Stomach.

- Assess how your emotions are impacted by your thoughts.

SPLEEN AND STOMACH

YOUR ENERGY GENERATORS

*EMOTIONS HAVE A STRONGER
EFFECT THAN FOOD ON OUR
BODIES...ON ONE LEVEL, YOU
ARE WHAT YOU EAT; AT A HIGHER
LEVEL, YOU ARE WHAT YOU THINK!*

–Grand Master Nan Lu

SPLEEN HIGHLIGHTS

PARTNER ORGAN:
Stomach

ELEMENT:
Earth

SENSE ORGAN:
Mouth

TISSUE ORGAN:
Muscles

EMOTION:
*Worry/
Overthinking*

SEASON:
Late Summer

COLOR:
Yellow

TASTE:
Sweet

STARTING THE WEEK

You're about to begin Week 4, the program's half-way point. Turn your attention to all that you ask your body to digest: foods, emotions, experiences, information and much more. All of that processing takes energy. This week, we focus on the role of the Spleen/Stomach pair in supporting the body's digestion.

Have you ever felt so worried that you had an immediate urge to run to the bathroom? It's not a coincidence. Your emotions are tied to the energetic functioning of your organs. Notice when you feel bloated or experience stomach pains. What are you digesting?

THE IMPORTANCE OF THE SPLEEN/STOMACH

The Spleen and Stomach help you accumulate Qi through the foods you eat. The body draws on this acquired Qi for everyday activities. When your bank of acquired Qi runs low, the body draws from its inherited Qi, stored in the Kidney. Our goal is to learn how to acquire and manage Qi wisely. That's the secret behind Dragon's Way Qigong.

The proper functioning of the digestive system depends on the overall health of Spleen/Stomach function and its relationship with the Liver. With a healthy digestive system, you can acquire more Qi and better absorb the nutrients in your food. Your digestive system is your first line of defense. Excess emotions, like worry and anger, play a major role in unbalancing the digestive system.

WHAT THE SPLEEN/STOMACH CAN DO

The Spleen/Stomach is the body's daily energy generator. The Stomach receives foods and liquids and rots and ripens them. The Spleen then transforms this food matter into essence. This essence forms the foundation for healthy Qi and blood that nourishes the entire body. High-quality blood and Qi translates into overall immune health and longevity.

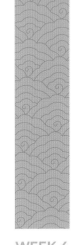

WEEKLY GOAL

Your digestive system processes food, emotions and your hectic lifestyle. My goal this week is to help you recognize where your processing is off-balance. Can you slow down, smooth out and help yourself easily digest every aspect of life?

–Grand Master Nan Lu

WHAT DOES IT LOOK LIKE WHEN THE SPLEEN/STOMACH DOES NOT FLOW SMOOTHLY?

- Worry and overthinking
- Weak or aching muscles
- Tendency to bruise easily
- Overweight, underweight
- Migraines (center of forehead)
- White coating on the tongue
- Bad breath
- Excess burping
- Lack of appetite
- Fatigue/insomnia
- Food allergies
- Menstrual bleeding: spotting
- Bloating or loose stools after eating

TUNE INWARD

Worry impacts your entire digestive process. What's on your mind? Write your thoughts below. Can you begin to let go little by little?

FIVE ELEMENT CONSCIOUSNESS FRAMEWORK

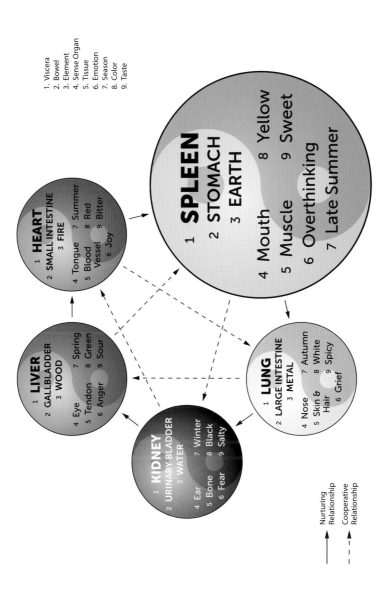

1. Viscera
2. Bowel
3. Element
4. Sense Organ
5. Tissue
6. Emotion
7. Season
8. Color
9. Taste

SPLEEN
1 SPLEEN
2 STOMACH
3 EARTH
4 Mouth
5 Muscle
6 Overthinking
7 Late Summer
8 Yellow
9 Sweet

HEART
1 HEART
2 SMALL INTESTINE
3 FIRE
4 Tongue
5 Blood Vessel
6 Joy
7 Summer
8 Red
9 Bitter

LIVER
1 LIVER
2 GALLBLADDER
3 WOOD
4 Eye
5 Tendon
6 Anger
7 Spring
8 Green
9 Sour

KIDNEY
1 KIDNEY
2 URINARY BLADDER
3 WATER
4 Ear
5 Bone
6 Fear
7 Winter
8 Black
9 Salty

LUNG
1 LUNG
2 LARGE INTESTINE
3 METAL
4 Nose
5 Skin & Hair
6 Grief
7 Autumn
8 White
9 Spicy

→ Nurturing Relationship
---- Cooperative Relationship

WEEK 4

RELATIONSHIPS

The Spleen/Stomach and Liver must support one another for good digestive health. If you find yourself with acid reflux or an overall feeling of "being stuck," it's a sign that the relationship between these organs is off-balance.

ELEMENT: EARTH

The Earth receives and accepts everything. Think of the Earth as the center of nurturing and absorption. This is the same relationship that the Spleen/Stomach has within the body.

SENSE ORGAN: MOUTH

The mouth is the opening gate to the outside of the body. If you have fresh breath, don't experience mouth sores and your gums don't bleed or swell, your body is showing signs of healthy Stomach function.

TISSUE ORGAN: MUSCLE

The muscles are the tissue organs associated with the Stomach. Strong, developed muscles are a sign of healthy Spleen/Stomach function.

EMOTION: WORRY/OVERTHINKING

Worry and overthinking are energy frequencies that can unbalance the partnership between the Spleen and Stomach.

SEASON: LATE SUMMER

Late Summer is the season when Earth's energies are transitioning from the sticky days of Summer to cooler Autumn weather. Summer fruits have reached their peak and Nature is rebalancing, preparing for a time of rest. Late Summer is a time to nourish our bodies with warming, freshly grown foods to support the digestive system.

COLOR: YELLOW

The color yellow has an energetic frequency that connects with the Spleen/Stomach. Wear yellow and eat warming foods and those grown in the Earth, such as carrots, sweet potatoes, ginger, turmeric and cinnamon, to support this organ system.

TASTE: SWEET

Sweet cravings are your body's way of communicating that your Spleen/Stomach Qi needs support. Try some mangoes, berries or watermelon. But if you're craving chocolate, go for it! Have a piece of dark chocolate and enjoy it 100%.

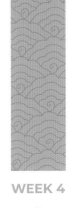

THE BODY NEVER LIES

MESSAGES FROM YOUR SPLEEN/STOMACH

How do you know if your Stomach Qi is talking to you? Are you aware of its messages?

YES NO

☐ ☐ **Do you crave sweets?**

☐ ☐ **Do you overthink situations?**

☐ ☐ **Do you get muscle aches or fatigue?**

☐ ☐ **Do you feel bloated after meals?**

If you answered "yes" to any of the above questions, follow these tips:

1. Amp up your Qigong practice!

2. Eat warm, cooked foods and soups daily.

3. Sing and dance. Allow your Qi to move!

DID YOU KNOW?

Food allergies are a symptom of energetic imbalance in your digestive system. Begin to support your digestive system by adding warming foods.

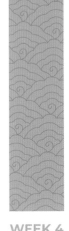

YOUR WEEKLY
ACTION PLAN

1. QIGONG PRACTICE: CREATING FLOW

Turn to the Qigong section. Practice movements 1–10 at least once per day and hold the last posture for about 15 minutes.

1. The Dragon's Toe Dance
2. The Dragon Kicks Forward
3. The Dragon's Twist
4. The Dragon's Punch
5. The Dragon Looks at Its Tail
6. The Dragon Taps Its Foot
7. Rocking the Baby Dragon
8. The Dragon Kicks Backward
9. The Dragon Rises from the Ocean
10. The Dragon Stands Between Heaven and Earth

WEEKLY CHALLENGE

As you practice number 9, imagine you are breathing in Universal good and pushing out everything you no longer need—fat, water, worry and stress.

–Grand Master Nan Lu

2. EATING-FOR-HEALING PLAN

When following the eating-for-healing plan, include some of these foods to further support your Spleen/Stomach function:

Chinese barley	Papaya
Lotus seed	Peanuts
Chinese red dates	Pumpkin
Red grapefruit	Ginger
Radishes	Cinnamon
Red grapes	Turmeric
Red apples	Fennel seeds
Sweet potato	Garlic
Mango	Black and white pepper

DID YOU KNOW?

Your Stomach loves warmth. Its function becomes unbalanced if you have a steady diet of cold, raw or processed foods and iced drinks. Nurture yourself by cooking vegetables before enjoying them and adding warming herbs and spices to your meals.

3. LIFESTYLE TIPS

1. This week is all about nurturing yourself. Do something spontaneous like going to a movie or going out to dinner by yourself.

2. Stop the worry, worry, worry! Try to see things from a different perspective. If you believe that everything happens for a reason, you will find it easier to let things go.

3. Continue reducing your exposure to computers and cell phones by taking more breaks during the day. A 15-minute break is the perfect time for a walk in Nature or an extra practice of *The Dragon Stands Between Heaven and Earth.*

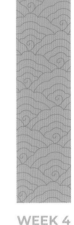

TRY THIS EXERCISE: MASSAGE

Massage the area from under your breastbone to above your navel to stimulate and soothe stomach function. Place one hand on top of the other and make 5 slow and gentle circles across the whole area. Repeat in the opposite direction.

CLOSING WORDS FOR WEEK 4

Are you feeling more energized or like a clean-up is still in process? Either way, keep going! The body requires a lot of Qi to change.

As you increase your Qi, your body, mind and Spirit come into a more harmonious communication. While this is the goal, deep healing can be accompanied by minor discomforts like loose stools or a skin rash. As your Qi begins to move freely, these discomforts will resolve naturally.

Push yourself a bit harder this week to follow the eating-for-healing plan and practice as often as possible. Make yourself the priority and you will reap the benefits. Your body has the wisdom to heal itself.

True change involves the willingness to see and accept our deepest selves.

–Grand Master Nan Lu

WEEK 4
JOURNAL

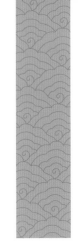

_____

_____

_____

_____

_____

_____

_____

_____

_____

_____

_____

_____

WEEK 4
JOURNAL

WEEK 4
JOURNAL

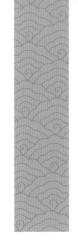

WEEK FIVE AT A GLANCE

THIS WEEK, WE'LL CONTINUE OUR FIVE ELEMENT JOURNEY TO LEARN ABOUT THE LUNG AND LARGE INTESTINE RELATIONSHIP. IN ADDITION, I'LL GUIDE YOU TO DO THE FOLLOWING:

WEEK 5

- Strengthen your Qigong movements with longer and more frequent practices.

- Prepare suggested foods that support the Lung and Large Intestine. You may find that the eating-for-healing plan is now an intuitive part of your daily routine.

- See yourself as valuable and let go of what holds you back. This is your time to shine!

LUNG
LET IT GO

*EVERY DAY IS AN OPPORTUNITY
TO DISCOVER YOURSELF AND TO
ALLOW YOUR INTUITION TO GROW.
CELEBRATE THE PROCESS EVEN
MORE THAN THE GOAL. AND THEN,
LET IT GO.*

–Grand Master Nan Lu

LUNG HIGHLIGHTS

PARTNER ORGAN:
Large Intestine

EMOTION:
Deep Sadness

ELEMENT:
Metal

SEASON:
Fall

SENSE ORGAN:
Nose

COLOR:
White

TISSUE ORGAN:
Skin

TASTE:
Spicy

STARTING THE WEEK

You're about to begin Week 5. What changes are you noticing? Often, this is the week when people begin to say how sensitive their taste buds have become. They can distinguish between fresh foods, processed foods and foods with chemicals and additives. Foods they once loved are no longer on their must-have list. This sensitivity will help you become aware of what your body needs at any given time. Note changes in your eating habits and the foods you now crave. Then reference the Five Element Consciousness Framework to see which organ is talking to you.

_____

_____

_____

THE IMPORTANCE OF THE LUNG

The Lung is known as the great distributor of Qi. Once the Stomach and Spleen complete the digestive process, the Spleen sends nutritive essence to the Lung. The Lung then decides how much Qi each organ receives and distributes it accordingly. This is a great example of the continual cooperative relationship within your body.

WHAT THE LUNG CAN DO

With every inhalation, the Lung helps your body communicate with the outside world. All of life depends on this action. The process of releasing from the inside-out is the duty of the Large Intestine. This duo must enjoy a cooperative relationship to allow the body to release and receive. The quality of your Lung Qi can be seen in the radiance of your skin. Dry, cracked skin and constipation are signs that the Lung and Large Intestine are not in balance.

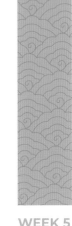

WEEKLY GOAL

My goal this week is to help you become more aware of what you're holding onto. Use the mantra "Let it go!" to support your change. Consider the message in the Tune Inward section that follows.

–Grand Master Nan Lu

WHAT DOES IT LOOK LIKE WHEN THE LUNG/LARGE INTESTINE DOES NOT FLOW SMOOTHLY?

- Persistent sadness
- Constipation
- Asthma, chronic cough
- Skin problems: dry skin, rashes, rosacea
- Fall allergies
- Bloated or puffy face
- Carpal tunnel, frozen shoulder
- Irregular heartbeat, heart palpitations
- Fatigue

TUNE INWARD

A Buddhist master and his student were walking toward the river when they heard a woman crying. She begged them to help her cross the river so she could reach her sick father. The monk carried her across the river. Then he said goodbye and continued on. The student became angry but kept silent for the rest of the journey. Many hours later, he exploded, "You carried a woman. This is forbidden!" "When did I do this?" asked the monk. "This morning!" the student shouted. "Ah," said the master. "I already put her down, but you've been carrying her all day long."

Use this story as a reminder to let it go.

FIVE ELEMENT CONSCIOUSNESS FRAMEWORK

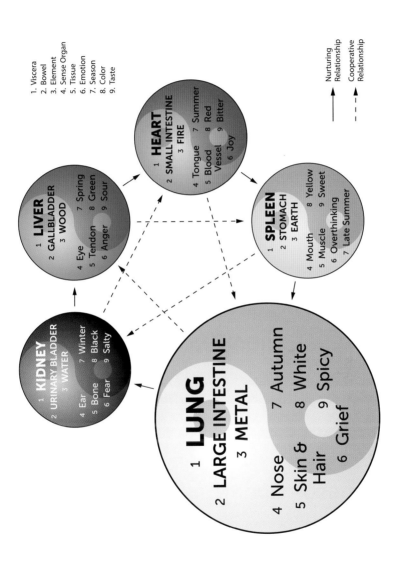

1. Viscera
2. Bowel
3. Element
4. Sense Organ
5. Tissue
6. Emotion
7. Season
8. Color
9. Taste

LIVER
2 GALLBLADDER
3 WOOD
4 Eye   7 Spring
5 Tendon 8 Green
6 Anger   9 Sour

HEART
1 SMALL INTESTINE
3 FIRE
2 ... 4 Tongue 7 Summer
5 Blood 8 Red
Vessel 9 Bitter
6 Joy

SPLEEN
2 STOMACH
3 EARTH
4 Mouth   8 Yellow
5 Muscle   9 Sweet
6 Overthinking
7 Late Summer

KIDNEY
2 URINARY BLADDER
3 WATER
4 Ear   7 Winter
5 Bone   8 Black
6 Fear   9 Salty

LUNG
2 LARGE INTESTINE
3 METAL
4 Nose   7 Autumn
5 Skin & 8 White
Hair   9 Spicy
6 Grief

⟶ Nurturing
Relationship

⇢ Cooperative
Relationship

WEEK 5

RELATIONSHIPS

The Lung and Large Intestine are partner organs. This pair continually supports one another in letting go and releasing. For example, if Lung Qi becomes weak, constipation may occur. Conversely, healthy Lung function will support healthy bowel function.

ELEMENT: METAL

The Metal element is related to the Lung. Metal is often thought of as cold, hard and powerful. Yet, Metal is also transformative! This shiny, precious element can be malleable and can even transform to liquid. Wearing jewelry is one sign you are associating with the Metal element.

SENSE ORGAN: NOSE

With every breath, the Lung draws in Universal Qi and connects the external world to the internal body. The nose is the sense organ associated with the Lung.

TISSUE ORGAN: SKIN

The skin is your largest organ. The Lung provides Qi and nourishment that directly supports the skin. Radiant, wrinkle-free skin is a sign that your Lung Qi is healthy. Keeping your skin covered in cold or windy weather helps support your Lung function.

EMOTION: DEEP SADNESS

Grief and sadness are the emotions associated with the Lung and Large Intestine. When these emotions are constant, the normal functioning of the Lung and Large Intestine will be impacted. Have you noticed that after a long crying spell, you begin to cough? That's the body's way of trying to rebalance itself.

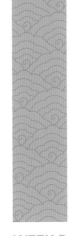

SEASON: FALL

Nature gives us a guide. Consider what happens during the Fall season. Trees drop their leaves to prepare for a period of rest. Follow Nature's lead—let go!

COLOR: WHITE

The color white resonates with the Lung. Wear white clothing and eat white foods, like almonds, white fungus and pears for additional support.

TASTE: SPICY

The taste that directly impacts the Lung is spicy. Spicy foods may make you sweat, which is how the body cools itself down. Notice when you crave spicy foods.

THE BODY NEVER LIES

MESSAGES FROM YOUR LUNG

Connect deeply with your body's messages. How does your skin look? Are there times when it's dry and itchy? During those periods, are you also constipated? Or does your skin have a nice glow? Begin to make connections.

Look back on the list of Lung/Large Intestine imbalances and note any that still apply to you. Remember, by increasing energy, the body will try to harmonize.

_____

_____

_____

DID YOU KNOW?

Do you continually wake up between 3 a.m. and 7 a.m.? If so, your Lung and Large Intestine system may be asking for more support. Study the Five Element Consciousness Framework for more information.

ACTION PLAN

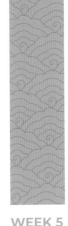

1. QIGONG PRACTICE: CREATING FLOW

Turn to the Qigong section. Practice movements 1–10 at least once per day and hold the last posture for 25 minutes.

1. The Dragon's Toe Dance

2. The Dragon Kicks Forward

3. The Dragon's Twist

4. The Dragon's Punch

5. The Dragon Looks at Its Tail

6. The Dragon Taps Its Foot

7. Rocking the Baby Dragon

8. The Dragon Kicks Backward

9. The Dragon Rises from the Ocean

10. The Dragon Stands Between Heaven and Earth

WEEKLY CHALLENGE

Take a mini break during your day and hold *The Dragon Stands Between Heaven and Earth* for an additional 10 minutes. Notice how this affects your mood and your energy level.

–Grand Master Nan Lu

2. EATING-FOR-HEALING PLAN

When following the eating-for-healing plan, include some of these foods to further support your Lung function:

Chili	Mushrooms
Almonds	Scallions
Bitter almonds	Chestnuts
Pears	Daikon radish
Persimmons	White sesame seeds
Honey	Lily bulb
White fungus	Mint
Horseradish	

DID YOU KNOW?

Although spicy is the taste that resonates with the Lung, certain foods on the above list—almonds, pears and honey—are chosen for their ability to support healthy Lung function. Try baking this trio for breakfast or a delicious treat!

3. LIFESTYLE TIPS

1. Stay indoors on windy days. Don't challenge Nature. Wind and cold are pathogens that can enter through the skin and lead to internal imbalances..

2. No more expensive face creams! Here's your secret to an ageless glow: The Lung disperses Qi to the tissues between the muscles and the skin. It also adds moisture to the skin. Include honey as part of your daily diet.

3. Keep it flowing. Regular bowel movements are a sign that your Lung and Large Intestine are in balance. As with the last tip, honey will help add moisture to your colon.

TRY THIS EXERCISE:

Close your eyes and slowly breathe in with your nose. When you breathe in, pull your stomach in. Then slowly breathe out from your mouth. When you breathe out, push your stomach out. Count each breath in and out as 1. After 5 breaths, breathe in slowly and deeply hold your breath for a slow count of 5. Exhale slowly. Repeat 2 or 3 times.

–Grand Master Nan Lu

CLOSING WORDS FOR WEEK 5

The only wrong way to practice is to not practice at all. Make your Qigong practice part of your everyday life. Use Qigong and your awareness of your body's innate wisdom to surround yourself with a sense of calm. During these few weeks, you are learning to communicate differently with your body and are allowing it to reawaken its natural healing abilities. Your body is a reflection of Nature. No matter the season, can you see yourself as part of Nature's cycles?

Before you begin the final week, assess the changes you are noticing within. Write them down below. Smile at the progress you are making.

> *Remember you are part of Nature.*
> *Remember you are part of the Universe.*
> *This energy—this wisdom—will be inside you forever.*
>
> *—Grand Master Nan Lu*

WEEK 5
JOURNAL

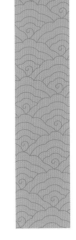

_____

_____

_____

_____

_____

_____

_____

_____

_____

_____

_____

_____

_____

WEEK 5
JOURNAL

WEEK 5

JOURNAL

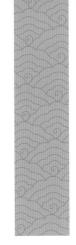

WEEK SIX AT A GLANCE

DURING WEEK 6, I'LL SHARE HOW TO READ MESSAGES FROM THE HEART AND SMALL INTESTINE ACCORDING TO THE FIVE ELEMENT CONSCIOUSNESS FRAMEWORK. IN ADDITION, I'LL GUIDE YOU TO DO THE FOLLOWING:

- Increase your Qigong practice to maximize your healing benefits. Notice how your movements have become more refined since the start of the program.

- Prepare suggested foods that support the Heart and Small Intestine.

- Learn additional lifestyle tips for happiness.

- Move forward after the 6-week program.

HEART
THE KING OF ALL ORGANS

*IF YOU WANT TO HEAL SOMEONE,
YOU HAVE TO FIRST HEAL
YOURSELF. IF YOU WANT TO LOVE
SOMEONE, YOU HAVE TO FIRST
LOVE YOURSELF. YOU CAN ONLY
GIVE SOMEONE WHAT YOU HAVE.
THE MORE YOU HAVE, THE MORE
YOU ARE ABLE TO GIVE.*

–Grand Master Nan Lu

WEEK 6

HEART HIGHLIGHTS

PARTNER ORGAN:
Small Intestine

EMOTION:
Joy

ELEMENT:
Fire

SEASON:
Summer

SENSE ORGAN:
Tongue

COLOR:
Red

TISSUE ORGAN:
Blood vessels

TASTE:
Bitter

STARTING THE WEEK

You're about to begin your final week in Dragon's Way Qigong. I hope you are deeply satisfied by the progress you've made in reacquainting yourself with your body's potential. You are changing from the inside-out. Remember, the invisible is more powerful than the visible. For sustainable change to happen, we must go to the invisible level of Qi.

You now have some tools to help you. But truly, you're just at the beginning of your journey! Continue to deepen your connection to Nature and your surroundings. Use this program again and again to build upon what you've begun. Reflect back on ways you have changed since the start of the program. Turn back to the Energy Inventory on page 24 and complete the "After" column.

THE IMPORTANCE OF THE HEART

In ancient Chinese tradition, the role of king was a sacred one. The king's ultimate mission was to take care of his people. He had to set an example by ruling with wisdom, compassion and love. His responsibility was to follow Natural Law and show how he is like the Tao itself—able to go with the flow, not worry and enjoy life.

The king was expected to let others manage the day-to-day duties of his kingdom. In the Five Element Consciousness Framework, this same concept applies to the Heart. Its duty is to remain peaceful and rely on the other organs to maintain balance. When other organs become seriously imbalanced, you may see signs of a Heart function disorder.

WHAT THE HEART CAN DO

The Heart is the connection between the physical world and the spiritual world. It is often said that once one opens the Heart, they experience true love. In love, there is no rational thinking, rather an intuitive way of being.

Imagine living your life fully open to receive the unconditional love of the Universe! Nothing and no one would bother you. You would be the king or queen of your own life.

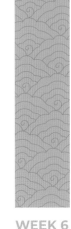

WEEKLY GOAL

My goal this week is to help you drop your mind and become more peaceful. With less mental activity, you can nurture the Heart and your innate creativity. You can connect with the limitless Tao only through the Heart, never the mind.

–Grand Master Nan Lu

WHAT DOES IT LOOK LIKE WHEN THE HEART/SMALL INTESTINE DOES NOT FLOW SMOOTHLY?

- Insomnia, difficulty sleeping

- Excess perspiration

- Pale complexion

- Pale, dark or cracked tongue

- Dry mouth

- Bright yellow urine

- Nightmares

- Poor digestion

- Lack of energy

- Depression, anxiety, panic attacks

- Irregular heartbeat

TUNE INWARD

All too often, we follow our daily schedule and forget to listen to the ultimate guiding source —the Heart. The Heart wants peace. Use your Qigong practice to balance your emotions and sharpen your intuition. Slow your body down so it can serve you more efficiently. Then you will be deeply honoring yourself.

FIVE ELEMENT CONSCIOUSNESS FRAMEWORK

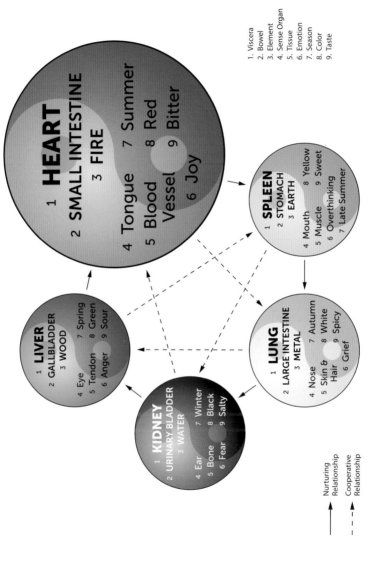

HEART
1 HEART
2 SMALL INTESTINE
3 FIRE
4 Tongue 7 Summer
5 Blood 8 Red
  Vessel 9 Bitter
6 Joy

SPLEEN
1 SPLEEN
2 STOMACH
3 EARTH
4 Mouth 8 Yellow
5 Muscle 9 Sweet
6 Overthinking
7 Late Summer

LIVER
1 LIVER
2 GALLBLADDER
3 WOOD
4 Eye 7 Spring
5 Tendon 8 Green
6 Anger 9 Sour

LUNG
1 LUNG
2 LARGE INTESTINE
3 METAL
4 Nose 7 Autumn
5 Skin & 8 White
  Hair 9 Spicy
6 Grief

KIDNEY
1 KIDNEY
2 URINARY BLADDER
3 WATER
4 Ear 7 Winter
5 Bone 8 Black
6 Fear 9 Salty

1. Viscera
2. Bowel
3. Element
4. Sense Organ
5. Tissue
6. Emotion
7. Season
8. Color
9. Taste

→ Nurturing
   Relationship
- - - Cooperative
   Relationship

RELATIONSHIPS

The Heart and Small Intestine work together to support all of the organs. The Heart is like the conductor of an orchestra. When all organs communicate in harmony, the Heart plays a beautiful symphony.

ELEMENT: FIRE

Fire is the element related to the Heart. Fire is vibrant and powerful. While it has the ability to destroy, it can also transform.

SENSE ORGAN: TONGUE

The tongue is the sense organ associated with the Heart. Colors and patterns that appear on the tongue help traditional Chinese medicine practitioners identify certain organ function disorders. Here's a map of the tongue:

> Heart: tip of the tongue
>
> Lung: just behind the tip and across the tongue
>
> Liver: sides of the tongue
>
> Kidney: back (toward the root) of the tongue
>
> Spleen/Stomach: center of the tongue

TISSUE ORGAN: BLOOD VESSELS

The Heart is responsible for the overall health of the blood vessels and the circulation of blood.

EMOTION: JOY

The Heart is associated with joy and love. Both support the creativity that happens when the Heart's energy is open and free-flowing.

SEASON: SUMMER

Summer is the season associated with the Heart. The fiery heat of Summer forces us to rest to allow the body time to cool down. It's also the time of year to enjoy Nature's show of colors. Enjoying cooling watermelon and other luscious summer fruits helps you connect to the abundance of Summer.

COLOR: RED

Red is a vibrant color that attracts a lot of attention or that says you are in charge. Some days you might be drawn to wearing this color. Notice how you feel.

TASTE: BITTER

Bitter foods resonate with the Heart. Give broccoli rabe and bitter melon a try this week.

THE BODY NEVER LIES

MESSAGES FROM YOUR HEART

As King of the organs, the Heart houses the Shen, or spirit. The Shen encompasses all mental, emotional and spiritual aspects of each person. TCM's definition of the mind includes aspects of consciousness, intelligence and thinking, memory and sleep, emotions and various aspects of the soul. Most mental and sleep problems can be traced straight to the source—unbalanced Heart Qi.

DID YOU KNOW?

Your face is a mirror of your emotions. Look in the mirror and notice your facial expressions. Do your facial muscles look tight or are they relaxed? Smile at yourself. Now deeply smile. Feel the difference between the two. Practice this until you feel a smile that can connect with your Heart. See if you can watch your face and feelings transform.

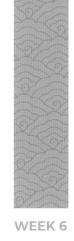

YOUR WEEKLY
ACTION PLAN

1. QIGONG PRACTICE: CREATING FLOW

Turn to the Qigong section. Practice movements 1–10 at least once per day and hold the last posture for 30 minutes.

1. The Dragon's Toe Dance

2. The Dragon Kicks Forward

3. The Dragon's Twist

4. The Dragon's Punch

5. The Dragon Looks at Its Tail

6. The Dragon Taps Its Foot

7. Rocking the Baby Dragon

8. The Dragon Kicks Backward

9. The Dragon Rises from the Ocean

10. The Dragon Stands Between Heaven and Earth

WEEKLY CHALLENGE

Real love comes from your Heart, not your mind. Train your mind to be silent. Sit comfortably and close your eyes. Do not control your breathing, rather let it be. Take mini meditation breaks several times each day.

–Grand Master Nan Lu

2. EATING-FOR-HEALING PLAN

When following the eating-for-healing plan, include some of these foods to further support your Heart function:

Broccoli rabe

Bitter melon

Watermelon

Plum tomatoes

Endive

Dandelion greens

Kale

Radicchio

Arugula

Apricots

Escarole

Berries

DID YOU KNOW?

Watermelon has a cool essence, so it can help cool down the body, relieve thirst and help the body release toxins. Used topically on the skin, watermelon is very effective for overexposure to the sun.

3. LIFESTYLE TIPS

1. Watch a funny movie. A good laugh will change your mood and stimulate your entire being.

2. Stop overworking the body! Sweating can be a sign that the Heart is overheated. Instead of running on a treadmill, practice Qigong.

3. Don't take yourself too seriously! Follow your Heart's lead and enjoy your life.

PEACEFUL BOOST

The palms of your hands connect to the Heart. By placing your palms together and closing your eyes, you will connect to messages of inner peace. For thousands of years, people have put their hands together in a prayer position to connect to a higher source. Use this posture to connect to that consciousness.

CLOSING WORDS FOR WEEK 6

I like to think of the initial 6 weeks as an awakening to a new journey. Don't stop here! You've opened the door to a path that can support you for the rest of your life.

Use the 10 Dragon's Way Qigong movements as your daily go-to. Practice each day to continue building your energy so the body has Qi to renew itself. Continue to follow your intuition in making healthy lifestyle and eating choices. Refer to the Five Element Consciousness Framework often. Your body will always remind you that you're on the right path by sending messages of balance.

If you are drawn to learning more about traditional Chinese medicine theories, I suggest reading *Traditional Chinese Medicine: A Natural Guide to Weight Loss That Lasts*. You can also visit tcmworld.org for additional information and programs and to view a list of certified Dragon's Way Qigong instructors in your area.

Good luck to you as you continue on this journey!

What you experience in the moment, from the pure pleasure of giving, is joy. What you feel after the fact, after the mind enters, is happiness. Joy is the inside coming out; happiness is the outside coming in.

–Grand Master Nan Lu

WEEK 6
JOURNAL

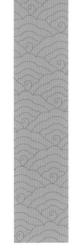

WEEK 6
JOURNAL

WEEK 6
JOURNAL

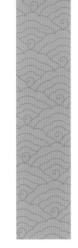

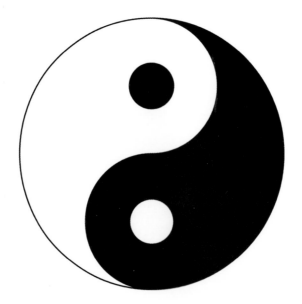

YIN/YANG: the symbol
of Universal Oneness

QIGONG

WHAT IS QIGONG & WHAT MAKES IT SO POWERFUL?

To understand Qigong, it's important to understand the role of Qi.

Qi is your life force. It's the energy that animates all things, including the human body. Your body has an innate wisdom to heal itself. When Qi flows freely, emotions are balanced, excess weight drops off and health issues resolve. Some call this a miracle. We know it's Qi!

To access the Qi level, we turn to Qigong practices. Qigong is the vehicle that allows us to accumulate and move energy in the body.

Based on ancient principles of traditional Chinese medicine, Qigong movements enable the body, mind and spirit to connect and communicate. Qigong functions like a telegraph system— transmitting and receiving code. This code is Qi, an energy with the ability to carry and convey information, intelligence and messages. We use Qigong practices as one of the major ways to support the body's constant desire for balance.

There are thousands of systems of Qigong practices. The Qigong system I teach dates back to the philosopher Laozi and is called *Wu Ming* Qigong, which when translated means "no name". It refers to the Universal state as it existed before the creation of Heaven and Earth. In ancient times, it was believed that the Universe was unlimited and energy was unlimited. Ancient philosophers believed we could connect to this unlimited source through energy practices, such as Qigong.

During your Dragon's Way Qigong experience you will practice 10 *Wu Ming* Qigong movements, arranged in such a way as to open your entire body to greater energy flow. From the first form, which begins with *The Dragon's Toe Dance,* the movements progress slowly up the entire body. Each posture supports the next and releases energy that may be stuck. Finally, the last movement, *The Dragon Stands Between Heaven and Earth,* will help you accumulate more Qi.

WHY DO YOU NEED TO ACCUMULATE QI?

In our busy lifestyle, we're continually using our natural resources of Qi. We try to accumulate Qi through sleep and eating, however that's not enough. If you're feeling overly tired, not sleeping, gaining weight, feeling stressed or experiencing other health issues, you are not acquiring enough daily Qi to maintain a healthy life. By adding these Dragon's Way Qigong practices, you're offering your body the ability to move and build Qi resources.

HOW TO PRACTICE
FOR THE BEST BENEFIT:

As with anything, consistent practice and dedication to deepening your skill will yield the highest benefits. Twenty minutes or more of daily practice can yield amazing results that you never thought possible. There are no special breathing techniques and special clothing is not necessary.

Watch the practice video. Start slowly, following the motion of each movement. Allow your body to feel the movements deeply within. As time progresses, you will find that your Qigong practice becomes more refined. Most people experience bursts of energy and feel their "foggy" mind drop away. Their internal Qi is waking up!

Follow the weekly guide, practicing the suggested movements for each week. Try to practice each for as long as you can. Add an additional practice whenever you have time. If you have a stressful day, hold the last posture for additional support.

DRAGON'S WAY QIGONG
MOVEMENTS

1. THE DRAGON'S TOE DANCE

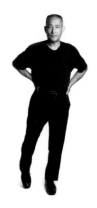

Place your hands on your lower back. Stand with your feet shoulder-width apart. Raise your left heel up and bend your knee. Your weight should be on the ball of your foot. Slowly rotate your left leg outward. Make sure your ankle, knee and hip joints turn together.

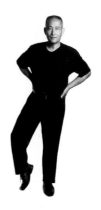

Count slowly: 1-2-3-4; 2-2-3-4; 3-2-3-4; 4-2-3-4; 5-2-3-4; 6-2-3-4; 7-2-3-4; 8-2-3-4. Complete 3 sets on your left side. Then repeat on the right side. Use this counting pattern for movements 1-8.

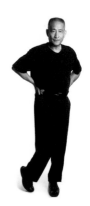

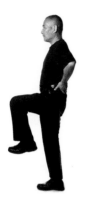

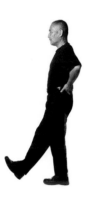

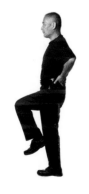

2. THE DRAGON
KICKS FORWARD

Place your hands on your lower back. Stand with your feet shoulder-width apart. Raise your left foot and kick forward gently with your heel, flexing your toes backward. Feel this stretch through the back of your leg. Relax your foot and bring it back so it is parallel with the floor. Gently lower your foot without touching the floor. Complete 3 sets, following the established counting pattern. Then repeat on the right side.

If you are unsteady, hold onto a chair for support. As your Qi increases, it will be easier to find your balance.

3. THE DRAGON'S TWIST

Place your hands on your lower back. Shift your weight to your right side and raise your left heel. Twist and allow your left hip bone to come forward. Be sure to keep your gaze forward. In this gentle swinging motion, your whole body twists from one side to the other. Complete 3 sets, following the established counting pattern.

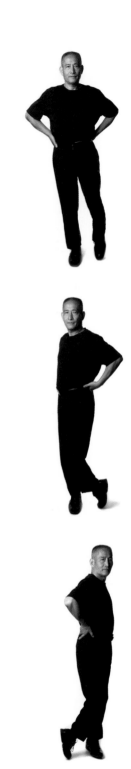

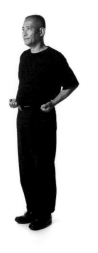

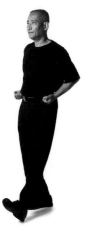

4. THE DRAGON'S PUNCH

Stand with your feet shoulder-width apart. Step forward in a gentle motion with your left foot, making sure your heel comes down first. As you step forward, gently punch your right hand forward. Twist your fist so that your fist "eye" points downward. Alternate with your right foot and left arm, punching in the same way. Complete 3 sets, following the established counting pattern.

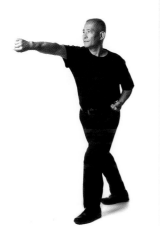

5. THE DRAGON LOOKS AT HIS TAIL

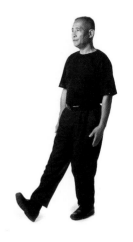

Stand with your feet shoulder-width apart. Step forward with your left leg. In the same motion, extend your right arm backward with your palm turned up. Turn your head and slowly look back toward your right palm. Alternate with the right leg and left arm, following the established counting pattern.

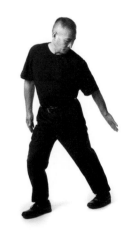

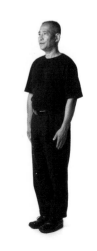

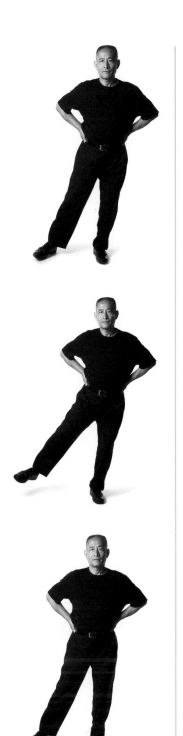

6. THE DRAGON TAPS HIS FOOT

Stand with your feet shoulder-width apart. Shift your weight to your left side. Stretch your right leg out to the side, lift it up a few inches and hit the inside of your right foot against the floor. Complete 3 sets, following the established counting pattern. Then repeat this movement with the left leg.

7. ROCKING THE BABY DRAGON

Stand with your feet shoulder-width apart. Bend your arms so that your fingers are pointing toward each other, palms facing up. Leaving a little space between your fingertips, slowly rock your arms to the left side while looking at your left elbow. Then bring your hands back to center before rocking your arms to the right side. Continue this motion, alternating left to right as you count. Complete 3 sets, following the established counting pattern.

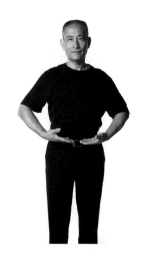

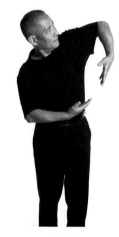

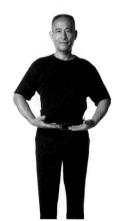

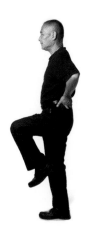

8. THE DRAGON
KICKS BACKWARD

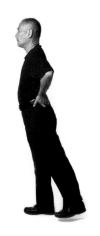

Place your hands on your lower back. Stand with your feet shoulder-width apart. Raise your left foot and kick backward gently with your heel. As you kick backward, you should feel a stretch through the back of your leg. Relax your foot and bring it up so it is parallel with the floor. Gently lower your foot without touching the floor. Complete 3 sets, following the established counting pattern. Then repeat on the right side.

If you are unsteady, hold onto a chair for support.

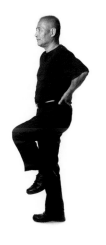

9. THE DRAGON RISES FROM THE OCEAN

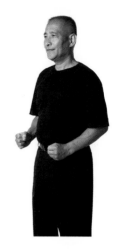

Stand with your knees bent, feet shoulder-width apart. Bend your elbows, holding tight fists at your sides. Breathe in deeply. When you breathe in, you are bringing Qi into your body. Exhale deeply. When you breathe out, imagine that you are pushing fat and water out of your body. Breathe in and out 20 times, counting 1 inhalation and exhalation as 1 breath. Do not rush your breathing.

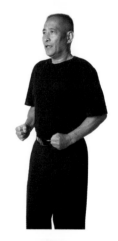

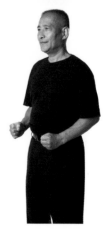

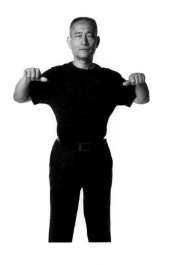

10. THE DRAGON STANDS BETWEEN HEAVEN AND EARTH

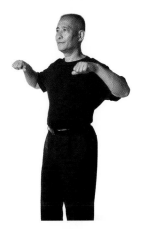

Stand with your knees slightly bent, feet shoulder-width apart. Raise your arms to chest level. Make fists with your thumbs pointing toward each other. Bend your elbows to bring your arms closer to your body. Close your eyes and imagine that you are the dragon standing between Heaven and Earth. Hold this position for at least 3 minutes to start; longer is better.

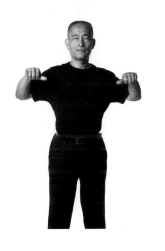

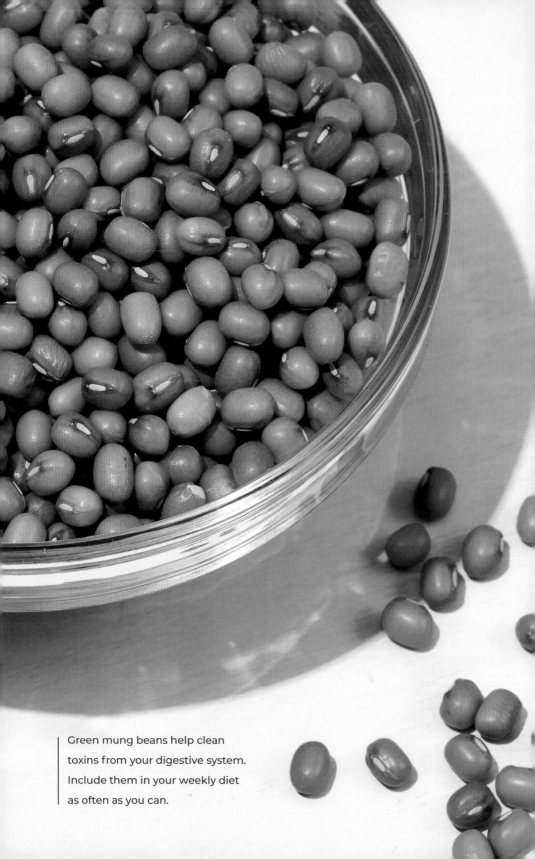

Green mung beans help clean
toxins from your digestive system.
Include them in your weekly diet
as often as you can.

EATING-FOR-HEALING PLAN

This eating-for-healing plan was developed with a healthy digestive system in mind. The digestive system must be able to receive the foods you eat, efficiently break them down and digest them before transforming your meal into usable Qi for the body. This process is often compromised by our modern-day eating style of salads and cold drinks.

As a general rule, try to eat foods that are slightly cooked or warmed. A steady diet of salads adds a cold essence to the digestive system, compromising its ability to be energy efficient. The body draws on excess energy to warm up raw food before beginning the digestive process.

By tweaking your diet to include more warming foods, your digestive system and your overall energy will improve in a short period of time. Eating in this manner will allow the digestive system to rest and to ultimately absorb the essence of the foods you eat.

The eating-for-healing plan in this program is primarily plant-based, encouraging fresh fruits, vegetables, nuts and occasionally, fish.

To gain the most out of the 6-week program, follow these guidelines as closely as possible.

Do not worry about cheating or falling off the wagon. Often, I hear people say, "I cheated. I didn't follow the diet!" This is not a diet, rather a style of eating that I think you will find easy to follow as the weeks progress.

If you have a particular craving, honor the craving and enjoy it 100%.

BEGIN YOUR NEW STYLE OF EATING

During the first week, reduce or eliminate bread, meat and dairy as best you can. These foods require more Qi to digest and I'd rather you use your Qi for healing. If you occasionally crave any of these foods, eat them! For example, adding 2 eggs weekly is fine as is having an occasional 1/2 cup of rice. As your eating style changes and lightens, you will feel the difference.

Be sure to cook or blanch your vegetables, even lettuce! Fruits can be eaten cooked or raw.

A simple way to curb overeating is to follow this rule: Eat until you are 70-80% full. Then become aware of why you are eating more: Are you truly hungry or are you eating for your eyes? Once you begin to eat lightly, you will find your hunger drops away and your food cravings change.

Here are a few more guidelines:

- Avoid fried and barbecued foods.

- Avoid drinking ice-cold fluids.

- Eat more soups.

- Eat nuts that are roasted or toasted.

- Eat your heaviest foods only in the morning or early afternoon.

- Eat fruits for lunch and vegetables for dinner.

- Drink only when you're thirsty.

- Drink more tea.

- Try to eat dinner before 7:00 P.M.

Select foods from the following list and add others that you enjoy. Dragon's Way Qigong is not about food restrictions, it's simply a style of eating that brings balance and harmony back to the body.

Once you have had a chance to review the list, take a look at the recipes that follow. Shop for your favorite foods and begin to develop your new style of eating.

SUGGESTED FOODS

Fruits:

- Apricots
- Berries of all kinds
- Dates
- Kiwis
- Lemons
- Mangoes
- Oranges
- Papayas
- Pears
- Persimmons
- Plum tomatoes
- Prunes
- Red Apples
- Red Grapefruits
- Red Grapes
- Strawberries
- Tangerines
- Watermelon

Vegetables:

- All greens
- Arugula
- Avocados
- Bamboo shoots
- Broccoli
- Broccoli rabe
- Carrots
- Cauliflower
- Celery
- Corn
- Dandelion
- Eggplant
- Escarole
- Fennel
- Green/Red peppers
- Kabocha squash
- Peas
- Radish
- Scallions
- Seaweed (all kinds)
- Snow peas
- Spinach
- Squash
- String beans

All spices, but especially these:

- Black and white pepper
- Black and white sesame seeds
- Chili pepper
- Cilantro
- Cinnamon
- Cloves
- Garlic
- Ginger
- Mint
- Mushroom seasoning
- Salt

All nuts, but especially these:

- Almonds
- Cashews
- Chestnuts
- Peanuts
- Pine nuts
- Walnuts

Oils:

- Avocado oil
- Olive oil
- Safflower oil
- Sesame oil
- Soy sauce
- Walnut oil

Other Suggestions:

- Bee pollen
- Honey
- Lotus
- Mushrooms
- Tea

SAMPLE MEALS

Here are some meal suggestions to help you get started. You can find these recipes and many more on tcmworld.org.

Breakfast:

Barley Cereal with Berries and Peanuts

Honey Baked Pears Compote

Mung Bean Cereal

Fresh Watermelon with Walnuts

Warm Nut Bowl with Raisins and Cranberries

Lunch:

Avocado Salad

Veggie Saute

Light Fish Soup

Bean Burger

Arugula Frittata

Dinner:

Roasted Eggplant with Pine Nuts

Tomato Chick Pea Salad

Kabocha Soup and Roasted Greens

Baked Fish with Dill

Roasted Vegetable and Daikon Radish Soup

SAMPLE RECIPES

Here's a sampling of some of our favorite recipes.

NURTURING TEA

Add 7-8 slices of fresh ginger, 1 juiced lemon (add skin if organic) and 1-2 tablespoons of honey to 1 quart of boiling water. Make a large pot and drink throughout the day.

REFRESHER TEA

Add fresh mint leaves or 2 mint tea bags to 3 cups boiling water. Let steep 5 minutes. Add the juice of 1/2 lemon and honey, to taste. For a richer taste, add lemon zest.

DANDELION TEA

Add 1 bunch of dandelion greens to a large pot of boiling water. Cover the pot and let simmer for 20 minutes. Discard the greens and sweeten the tea with brown sugar or honey, to taste. Drink throughout the day to cleanse your body.

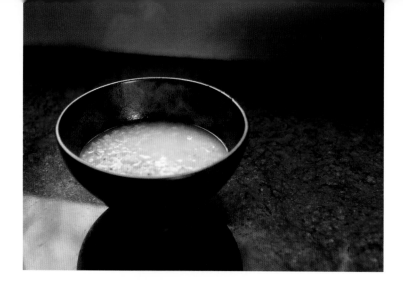

CHINESE BARLEY CEREAL

5 cups boiling water

1 cup rinsed barley

Add barley to the boiling water.

Stir and lower the heat to a simmer.

Cook covered for 20 minutes or until the water is absorbed.

TIP: The water tends to absorb quickly. Keep an eye on the barley, adding more water if needed to avoid burning.

Add your favorite spices, berries or nuts for variety.

Recent research has shown that barley cereal contains many anti-cancer properties. We love this cereal and suggest you enjoy it multiple times per week.

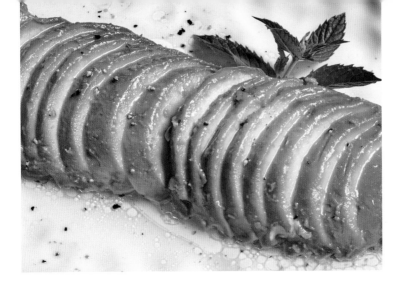

SLICED AVOCADO WITH LEMON DRESSING

2 ripe avocados

2 Tablespoons extra virgin olive oil

2 Tablespoons freshly squeezed lemon juice

sea salt, to taste

freshly ground pepper, to taste

Halve avocados lengthwise and remove the pits. Use a large spoon to scoop out the flesh.

Slice the fruit into wedges and place on a serving platter.

Drizzle with olive oil & lemon juice. Season with salt and pepper.

Serve at room temperature.

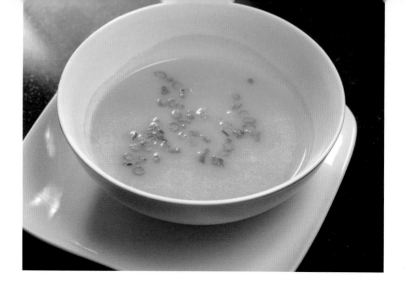

KABOCHA SQUASH SOUP

1/2 Kabocha squash, cubed

1 teaspoon salt

1 teaspoon mushroom seasoning

1 teaspoon butter

2 scallions, diced

Bring 1 quart of water to a boil. Add the kabocha squash and salt. Cook for 15 minutes. Add the mushroom seasoning. Then use an immersion blender to puree the squash to your desired consistency.

Add the butter and stir until melted.

Spoon into a bowl and top with the diced scallions.

TIP: Cut the skin off of the squash before chopping. If the skin is too thick, chop the squash in half and bake it, cut side down on a cookie sheet at 375 degrees for about 30 minutes. Then scoop out the flesh and add it to the boiling water.

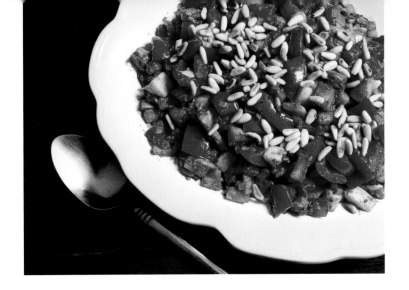

ROASTED EGGPLANT WITH PINE NUTS

1 small eggplant

5 plum tomatoes, chopped

1 spring garlic bulb or scallion, diced

2 Tablespoons pine nuts roasted

Salt and pepper, to taste

1 Tablespoon olive oil

Juice from 1/3 fresh lemon

Cut the eggplant into wedges. Salt the wedges and let them sit for 20 minutes. Then rinse the wedges and pat them dry.

Place the eggplant wedges in a baking dish. Top with tomatoes, garlic, pine nuts and salt and pepper, to taste. Drizzle with olive oil.

Bake, loosely covered, at 350 degrees for about 45 minutes.

Remove from the oven and squeeze the fresh lemon juice over the top. Serve warm.

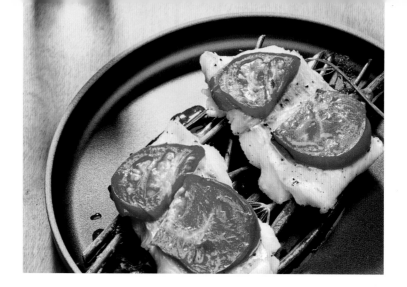

BAKED FISH WITH DILL

1/2 pound white fish fillets (cod, halibut)

1/4 teaspoon salt

1/4 teaspoon mushroom powder

1/4 cup olive oil

5-6 long stalks fresh dill

1 scallion, cut in 1/2 inch pieces

1 vine-ripened or plum tomato, sliced

Dash of wine

Sprinkle salt and mushroom powder on fish. Let sit 5 minutes.

Coat the bottom of an ovenproof pan with about 1 Tablespoon olive oil and a few sprigs of dill.

Place the fish in the pan. Garnish with remaining dill, scallion and tomato slices.

Add a splash of wine, then drizzle the remaining oil over the fish.

Bake in a preheated oven at 425 degrees for 15 minutes or until the fish flakes easily with a fork.

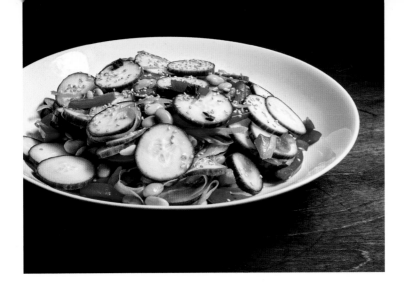

ASIAN CUCUMBER SALAD

3 seedless cucumbers, thinly sliced

1 red bell pepper, sliced

1 carrot, shredded

1 cup edamame, shelled

Toasted sesame seeds for garnish

DRESSING:

3/4 cup rice wine vinegar

1/4 cup water

2 Tablespoons sugar

1 teaspoon salt

2 Tablespoons cilantro, chopped

Add the vegetables and edamame to a large bowl. Mix.

Add all dressing ingredients to a small bowl. Whisk to combine.

Pour the dressing over the vegetables and toss to coat. Refrigerate for at least 1 hour. Toss again before serving.

Garnish with toasted sesame seeds.

This recipe is included in the program even though it contains raw vegetables. Are you wondering why? The vinegar breaks down the cold essence of the raw vegetables, making them easier to digest.

"IF YOU BELIEVE THAT THE BODY HAS THE ABILITY TO HEAL ITSELF, THEN TRUST THAT IT ALSO KNOWS WHAT IT NEEDS TO FIND BALANCE. FOLLOW YOUR FOOD CRAVINGS AND LISTEN TO YOUR BODY, NOT YOUR MIND."

–Grand Master Nan Lu

ADDITIONAL
NOTES

ADDITIONAL
NOTES

_____

_____

_____

_____

_____

_____

_____

_____

_____

_____

_____

_____

_____

ADDITIONAL
NOTES